Tantric Sex Bible

A Comprehensive Guide on How to Practice Tantra's Intimate Form of Sex and Tantric Sex Techniques to Enhance Your Connection with Your Partner

Cheryl Bach

Tantric Sex Bible

Publisher: IntimateInk Press

Email: intimateinkpress@gmail.com

This book is a work of nonfiction intended for informational purposes only. The content of this book is based on the author's research, knowledge, and experience, and it is provided with the understanding that the author and publisher are not engaged in rendering legal, medical, or professional advice. The information in this book is not a substitute for professional guidance or assistance. Readers should consult with relevant professionals for advice and assistance regarding their specific situations. The author and publisher disclaim any liability for any loss or risk, personal or otherwise, which is incurred as a consequence, directly or indirectly, of the use and application of any of the contents of this book.

Cover design by IntimateInk Press

Interior layout and design by IntimateInk Press

Printed in USA

Fonts: Google fonts

Image: Freepik.com. This cover has been designed using assets from Freepik.com

First Edition: 2024

Distributed by Amazon.com, Inc.

Cheryl Bach

Table of Contents

TABLE OF CONTENTS 3

INTRODUCTION 7

Benefits of Practicing Tantric Sex in Your Intimate Relationship 8

Overview of the Content and Structure of the Book..........10

CHAPTER 1 ....**13**

Foundation of Tantra...13

The History of Tantra..14

The Philosophy of Tantra 15

Integrating Tantra into Daily Life..............................16

CHAPTER 2 ....**21**

The Art of Sensual Touch 21

Understanding the Power of Touch in Tantric Sex............21

Different Types of Touch and Their Effects on the Senses 22

Techniques for Enhancing and Focusing Touch..................24

CHAPTER 3..**27**

BREATHWORK 27

Breathing Techniques for Increasing Intimacy and Pleasure...27

Synchronizing Breath with Your Partner.........................29

CHAPTER 4..**33**

THE POWER OF MEDITATION AND CONCENTRATION 33

Understanding the Role of Meditation and Focus in Tantric Sex..33

Different Types of Meditation Techniques..........................34

Importance of Concentration and How to Enhance It.....36

Incorporating Meditation and Concentration into Tantric Sex...38

CHAPTER 5..**43**

TANTRA'S SEXUAL PRACTICES...43

The Basics of Tantra's Sexual Practices.............................43

The Kama Sutra...44

Yoni Massage...45

Techniques for Increasing Pleasure and Connection.......46

Benefits of Sexual Practices in Achieving Higher States of Consciousness...47

The Importance of Consent.................................48

CHAPTER 6...**51**

INCORPORATING TANTRA INTO YOUR RELATIONSHIP.....................51

*How to Approach Discussing Tantra with Your Partner*51

Introducing Tantra into Your Intimate Relationship.......54

Building Trust and Communication in Your Relationship through Tantra...56

Embracing Spirituality in Your Relationship through Tantra...58

CHAPTER 7...**63**

ADVANCED TANTRA TECHNIQUES.................................63

Advanced Techniques.................................63

Navigating Challenges and Setbacks in Your Practice....66

Advancing Your Spiritual and Intimate Connection.........67

CHAPTER 8...**69**

MAINTAINING YOUR TANTRIC PRACTICE.................................69

Tips for Continuing to Practice Tantra in Your Everyday Life...69

How to Incorporate Tantra into Long-Term Relationships 73

Navigating Changes in Your Relationship through Continued Practice 74

CHAPTER 9 ....**77**

CONCLUSION 77

Introduction

Tantra is an ancient practice that originated in India over 5,000 years ago. In Sanskrit, Tantra means "weave" or "woven together". It's a spiritual practice that encompasses all aspects of life, including sexuality, and aims to help individuals achieve enlightenment by connecting with their divine essence.

Tantric Sex involves intimate sexual connection that involves the body, mind, and spirit. It encourages individuals to embrace and celebrate their sexuality while providing a means to further empower their spiritual selves.

Benefits of Practicing Tantric Sex in Your Intimate Relationship

There are numerous benefits to practicing Tantric Sex in your intimate relationship.

Some of these benefits include:

Emotional Connection - Tantric Sex encourages emotional intimacy between partners. By focusing on the present moment and being physically present with one another, partners can connect with each other on a deeper level emotionally. This emotional closeness is essential in building trust and intimacy.

Mindfulness and Presence - Tantric Sex emphasizes the importance of mindfulness and presence during intimate moments. Rather than being distracted by past or future thoughts, it encourages partners to be fully present and attentive to their partner's needs.

Increased Pleasure - By embracing your sexuality and exploring new methods of sexual pleasure, Tantric Sex can lead to increased physical pleasure and intensity of orgasms.

Higher Spiritual Connection - Tantric Sex seeks to connect individuals with their spiritual selves. By embracing sexuality as a part of the spiritual journey, individuals can develop a deeper understanding of themselves and their partners.

Extended Sexual Experience - Tantric Sex is not just about the moment of orgasm but focuses on the journey towards it. By exploring physical touch and sensations, partners can extend the sexual experience and enjoy it for a longer period.

Improved Communication - Tantric Sex requires communication, trust, and respect between partners. By communicating their needs and desires and listening to their partner's needs, couples can strengthen their emotional connection and improve their sexual life.

Overview of the Content and Structure of the Book

The book, "Tantric Sex Bible: A Comprehensive Guide on How to Practice Tantra's Intimate Form of Sex and Tantric Sex Techniques to Enhance Your Connection with Your Partner," is designed to help couples explore Tantric Sex as an intimate form of sexuality and reap its benefits.

The book starts with understanding tantra and its philosophy. This part provides a comprehensive overview of Tantra, its history, philosophy and how it relates to sexuality. It explains the various types of Tantra and how they can be applied to your intimate relationships.

We will also discuss Tantric Sex Techniques and Practices. In this section, you will learn the various Tantric Sex techniques, such as breathing techniques, guided meditations, and yoga practices that they can incorporate into their love life to enhance their connection and intensify their pleasure. It covers various aspects of foreplay, the importance of touch, different sexual positions, and much more.

And finally, we will discuss exploring sexual energies. This part of the book teaches couples how to awaken their sexual energy, increase their libido, and explore each other's bodies in new and exciting ways. It helps readers to understand the nature of sexual energy and how it can be harnessed to deepen their connection with their partner.

Welcome to the world of tantric sex, let's explore this aspect of our sexuality together.

Chapter 1

Foundation of Tantra

Tantra is a philosophy and practice that originated in ancient India over a thousand years ago. The term 'Tantra' is derived from Sanskrit and refers to the weaving and expansion of energy. Tantra is a way of life that combines spiritual practices with self-awareness and introspection.

Tantra is not just limited to sexual practices but also involves other aspects of life such as yoga, meditation, ritual, and spirituality. Tantra is a path towards awakening and realizing your true self through techniques and practices that connect you to the divine.

The History of Tantra

Tantra has been practiced for centuries throughout South Asia and beyond. Its roots can be traced back to ancient India, where it was a practice of self-realization and spirituality. It later spread to Tibet, China, Japan, and other parts of the world in various forms.

Tantra was often practiced in secret due to societal norms and taboos regarding sexuality. It was considered a taboo subject and was often misunderstood and misrepresented by those who were not familiar with its true purpose and practices.

In modern times, Tantra has become more widely known and accepted as a path to spiritual and sexual awakening. There are now many Tantra teachers and practitioners offering workshops and training programs around the world.

Cheryl Bach

The Philosophy of Tantra

At the core of Tantra is the belief that everything in the universe is interconnected and that humans are capable of transcending this connection through spiritual practices. Tantra encourages individuals to embrace their true selves, accepting all parts of themselves without judgement or shame.

Tantric philosophy emphasizes the importance of pleasure and connection as a means of awakening the senses and also teaches that one should approach life with an open heart and an open mind, embracing the present moment and experiencing it fully.

Tantric philosophy also involves balancing the masculine and feminine energies within oneself, recognizing that these energies are not limited to gender but are present in all individuals. This balance is essential for cultivating a sense of wholeness and completeness.

Integrating Tantra into Daily Life

Tantric practices are not limited to sexuality and can be integrated into one's daily life in various ways. Tantra encourages individuals to lead a balanced life, incorporating practices such as yoga, meditation, and mindfulness into their daily routine.

Here are some tips to get started:

Cultivate Awareness - Mindfulness during daily activities is essential for tantric practice. Being present, breathing consciously, and paying attention to your senses will enhance the experience.

Practice Sensual Touch - Discover ways to connect with others through sensual touch. It nurtures intimacy, improves communication, and encourages emotional expression.

Meditate Regularly - Meditation helps to calm the mind, focus on intention, and foster the growth of spiritual energy. Developing this practice daily provides peace, clarity, and balance.

Embrace your sexuality - Embracing sexual desire and curiosity can deepen sensual awareness and connection. Honoring intimacy in all forms, frees from negative patterns and liberates one unlimited pleasure.

Appreciate & Embrace the Divine Feminine and Masculine - Both energies bring balance to daily life, which is essential for personal and spiritual growth. Integrating both energies fosters a deeper appreciation of our own unique qualities, as well as those of others.

Experiment with Energy Work - Exploring energy work like Qigong or Reiki, teaches the body the releases and channels universal energy. Practicing regularly helps to harmonize the mind, elevate spiritual existence and improve health.

Practice Self-Love - Embrace the beauty of your imperfections and forgive yourself through self-love practices. Supplement yourself with patience, acceptance, and understanding. Creating a stronger self-love means you radiate more externally too.

Connect with Nature - Spend time connecting with the natural world, feeling its beauty and magnificence. Nature merges individual consciousness with the universal one, leading to a feeling of interconnection with all things. It is a powerful tool for grounding and centering, creating a space to reset.

Integrating the principles of Tantra into daily life is a journey of self-discovery and growth. Remember to be gentle with yourself during the process and embrace your inner beauty. The rewards of incorporating these practices into daily life are vast and enriching.

Chapter 2

The Art of Sensual Touch

The Art of Sensual Touch is a vital aspect of Tantric Sex. It is through touch that we can connect with our bodies, our partners, and the universal energy present in all things. In this chapter, we'll explore how touch can be a transformative tool for intimacy, connection and pleasure.

Understanding the Power of Touch in Tantric Sex

Tantric Sex is a practice where every touch is deliberate and mindful, from exploring intimate areas to just holding hands. It is through touch that we connect to the physical body, our emotions, and spiritual energy, which opens us up to heightened sensitivity and awareness while having sex.

The power of touch lies in its ability to take us on an intimate journey of both pleasure and healing. Touch serves not only as a physical pleasure but also as a form of emotional connection where consensual touch can trigger positive emotional responses and increase oxytocin levels in the body, creating a deeper sense of bonding and trust with your partner.

Different Types of Touch and Their Effects on the Senses

During Tantric Sex, different types of touch can be used to awaken our senses, providing us with varying experiences based on the type of touch we use.

Light Touch - It is a gentle, feather-like caress on the skin; it stimulates nerve endings on the skin's surface, enhancing our awareness of touch. This type of touch creates a subtle and relaxing experience which can add depth to intimate moments.

Firm Touch - It helps to regulate emotions and create grounding when feeling overwhelmed during intimate moments. It provides a sense of stability, grounding and balance. Firm touch can also be used as a warm-up for more intense touch later on.

Teasing Touch - It is used to create anticipation and heightened pleasure sensations before climax. This kind of touch can add excitement to intimate moments and prolong the duration of sexual pleasure.

Relaxing Touch - It helps to create a deeper sense of intimacy and connection with your partner during sex. Relaxing touch can be essential in creating a calm and peaceful atmosphere that allows both partners to connect on a deeper level.

Techniques for Enhancing and Focusing Touch

Here are some techniques you can use to enhance and focus touch during Tantric Sex:

Mindful Touch - Practicing mindfulness during sex helps maintain focus on every moment and sensation being felt. Being present and engaged in the moment connects us to our partner while allowing us to experience each touch fully.

Breathing Techniques - Slowing down our breathing allows us to relax our body and mind. Deep, slow breaths help control the pace of sexual activity while also increasing sensitivity levels during intimate moments.

Experimenting with Different Parts of The Body - Using different parts of the body like fingers, lips and even toes can add to the variety of sensations you feel during sex, creating exciting new experiences with your partner.

Warm Oil Massage - Sensual massages can be a wonderful way to connect intimately with your partner while also relaxing the body. Using warm oil can relieve tension in the muscles while also stimulating senses.

All in all, The Art of Sensual Touch is an essential aspect of Tantric Sex. By being mindful of our touch and experimenting with different types of touch, we can create deeper connections with our partners, leading to heightened levels of pleasure, trust, and intimacy during sex. Tantric Sex emphasizes the importance of touch as a transformative tool to increase awareness of our bodies and the energy surrounding us, leading us to a deeper sense of connection with our partners.

It is important to note that each partner may have different types of touch that they prefer, and open communication about each other's preferences can lead to more satisfying sexual experiences for both partners.

In Tantric Sex, touch is not solely focused on physical pleasure but aims to create a union between mind, body and spirit. Engaging in The Art of Sensual Touch can help you build better relationships, explore your sexual desires on a deeper level and establish a stronger emotional connection with your partner, ultimately leading to more pleasurable experiences during intimate moments.

Chapter 3

Breathwork

Breath is a powerful healer, and in Tantric Sex, it plays an important role. Breathing techniques help us to maintain focus on present sensations, create intimacy with our partners and increase pleasure during sex. Breathing is essential in activating our energies, helping us to move past any physical or emotional blocks that may hinder our enjoyment of intimate moments.

Breathing Techniques for Increasing Intimacy and Pleasure

Tantric Sex is a practice that engages all senses, and the breath is no exception.

Here are some breathing techniques that partners can engage in to enhance intimacy and pleasure:

Deep Breathing - Before engaging in sexual activities, taking deep breaths can calm your mind and help you connect with your body. Deep breathing allows oxygen to flow more freely in the bloodstream, helping to relax the body and create a sense of clarity, making it easier to focus on your partner and the present moment. Moreover, it helps to increase your body's sensitivity to touch by alerting the nervous system.

Circular Breathing - This is a technique in which you inhale and exhale in a circular rhythm, creating a flow of breath that is continuous. It helps to create an intense and uninterrupted connection with your partner, building intimacy while also increasing the level of pleasure experienced during sex.

Alternate Nostril Breathing - This is an ancient breathing technique used in yoga to balance the left and right hemispheres of the brain. The technique involves inhaling through one nostril while holding the other closed, then exhaling through the other nostril while blocking the other. It helps to create a sense of balance, making it easier for partners to experience deeper connections with each other during intimate moments.

Orgasmic Breathing - This technique involves synchronized breathing with your partner during sex to enhance pleasure and intimacy. It involves rhythmic breathing in a circular motion while engaging in sexual activities, such as stroking and embracing.

Synchronizing Breath with Your Partner

Synchronization of breath during intimate moments can be challenging for partners, but it's an essential aspect of Tantric Sex.

Here are some techniques that can help you to synchronize your breath with your partner:

Mindful awareness - During sexual activity, each partner must pay careful attention to their breathing patterns. They should observe the timing and depth of their breaths and try to match their breaths with each other.

Start slow - It's important to start slowly when learning how to synchronize breath with your partner. Focusing too much on deep breathing patterns may create an undesirable outcome. Therefore, start by simply breathing in sync with your partner and then slowly develop a rhythm.

Eye contact - Throughout sex, partners should maintain eye contact as they synchronize their breaths. This will help to establish a deep sense of connection while also enhancing the pleasurable sensations experienced during intimate moments.

Cheryl Bach

Verbal cues - Partners can use verbal cues to help synchronize their breaths during sexual activities. One partner can vocalize and count breaths or give instruction while the other mimics it.

By syncing breath during sex, the energy flow between partners increases, making sensations rich and erotic. It creates an intense sensory experience leading to deep connection and intimacy between partners.

To conclude, breathing techniques play a crucial role in Tantric Sex by enhancing emotional and physical connections between partners. This allows for a deeper understanding of our bodies and being present with oneself and one's partner during intimate moments. By syncing breaths, connections deepen simultaneously with sensations, which leads to intense and more pleasurable experiences.

Through practice, breathing techniques during Tantric Sex become automatic, leading to a more profound and a soulful sexual connection between partners. Engaging in Tantric Sex helps couples develop an awareness of their bodies and the surrounding energy, leading to a more fulfilling sexual life. By learning how to regulate and control breath, couples can take their intimacy to new heights, achieving a greater sense of physical, emotional and spiritual fulfillment.

Chapter 4

The Power of Meditation and Concentration

Understanding the Role of Meditation and Focus in Tantric Sex

Meditation is an essential part of tantric sex practice. It helps to calm your mind, focus on the present moment, and allow you to be more fully present and engaged during sex. When you're fully present, you'll become more aware of your body, your breath, and your sensations, which can lead to a deeper level of connection with your partner.

In tantric sex, meditation involves cultivating awareness, acceptance, and non-judgmental observation of your thoughts, feelings, and physical sensations. This can help you become more conscious of your body and enhance your ability to achieve deep relaxation and heightened sensitivity during sexual activity. When you incorporate meditation into your tantric sex practice, you'll be able to fully explore and enjoy your physical sensations, emotions, and intimacy with your partner.

Different Types of Meditation Techniques

Here are some different types of meditation techniques that can be used to improve your concentration and awareness during tantric sex:

Mindfulness Meditation - This is a type of meditation that involves focusing your attention on the present moment and becoming aware of your thoughts, feelings, and physical sensations without judgment or distraction. When practicing mindfulness meditation, you become an observer of your thoughts and feelings, which can help you cultivate mental clarity while avoiding distractions during intimate moments.

Loving-Kindness Meditation - Also known as 'Metta Meditation', this practice cultivates feelings of love, compassion, and kindness towards yourself and others. When engaging in loving-kindness meditation, you focus on visualizing love and kindness towards yourself and others. This type of meditation is beneficial for enhancing your overall well-being and developing positive emotions that can translate into deeper intimacy with your partner.

Chakra Meditation - According to Tantra, there are seven energy centers known as chakras located in the body. Chakra meditation involves focusing on each chakra center and visualizing a specific color and sound associated with it. This can help to balance your energy flow throughout your body and enhance your sexual energy.

Breath Awareness Meditation - Focusing on your breath is a common practice in many forms of meditation. In breath awareness meditation, you focus solely on your breathing to help calm your mind, deepen your relaxation, and enhance your connection with your partner during sex.

Importance of Concentration and How to Enhance It

Concentration is important in tantric sex because it helps you stay present and focused on the intimate moment with your partner. Without concentration, it becomes easy to get distracted and lose the connection with your partner, leading to unsatisfying sex.

Here are some tips on how to enhance your concentration during tantric sex:

Practice meditation daily - Meditation helps develop a disciplined mind that's more likely to focus and concentrate during intimate moments. Practicing meditation daily can help improve your overall concentration and mindfulness.

Remove distractions - During tantric sex, it's essential to remove all possible distractions, such as TV, phone calls, or anything else that may take your attention away from the intimacy. Turning off any electronic devices and putting them away can be helpful in ensuring zero distractions.

Use affirmations - Affirmations support a positive mindset that enhances concentration. Positive affirmations can help you remain focused on the present moment and in touch with your body and partner. Some examples of affirmations include "I am connected to my body," "I am present in this moment," or "I am fully focused on my partner."

Focus on your breath - Focusing on your breath can help anchor you in the present moment and prevent distractions. During intimate moments with your partner, continuously focus on your breath. When your mind starts to wander, gently bring it back to your breath.

Engage in Foreplay - Taking your time during foreplay can be an excellent way to increase concentration and intimacy. Touching your partner's entire body, kissing, and creating anticipation can help create a strong connection, leading to better concentration when engaging in intercourse.

By practicing these simple techniques, you can enhance your concentration, improve your mindfulness, and allow yourself to fully enjoy the intimate moments of tantric sex.

Incorporating Meditation and Concentration into Tantric Sex

Here are some ways to incorporate meditation and concentration techniques into your tantric sex practice:

Start with a meditation – Before engaging in sexual activity, take time to meditate for a few minutes. It can be helpful to close your eyes, focus on your breath, or tune-in to your body's physical sensations. This will help you become more present and focused before engaging in intimacy with your partner.

Focus on Breathing – Try focusing solely on your breathing during sex. Use deep breathing techniques to help calm your mind and body, bringing greater relaxation and heightened sensitivity.

Maintain Eye Contact - Intense eye contact, combined with deep breathing, can help increase intimacy and deepen the connection you have with your partner.

Use Mantras or Affirmations - Incorporating mantras or affirmations can help you stay connected and focused on the present moment during sex. You can silently repeat a word or phrase to yourself, such as "I am present," "I am connected to my partner," or any word/phrase that resonates with you.

Try Chakra Meditation - Chakra meditation can help increase energy flow during sex, making it a powerful practice to incorporate. Focus on each chakra center and visualize its corresponding color to help balance your energy and increase your pleasure.

Slow Down during Sex - Take your time during sex. Focus on the specific sensations that you are experiencing at the moment; notice the touch, sounds, smells, and movements. Practicing mindful sex will help you stay focused on the present moment.

Experiment with Multiple Positions - Try practicing tantric sex in different positions to enhance your connection with your partner. Experiment with positions that allow for deeper intimacy and eye contact.

By incorporating these meditation and concentration techniques into your tantric sex practice, you can deepen your connection with your partner and increase your overall satisfaction and pleasure. Remember to take your time, stay present, and focus on your breath and sensations.

Chapter 5

Tantra's Sexual Practices

The Basics of Tantra's Sexual Practices

Tantra's sexual practices involve using the sexual energy to achieve higher states of consciousness, which can lead to spiritual growth and enlightenment. This is done through the union of the masculine and feminine energies, known as Shiva and Shakti respectively.

The basis for any tantric practice begins with mindfulness and awareness. It's essential to be present in the moment, fully aware of the physical sensations that arise during sex. This helps prevent distractions and allows you to focus solely on the pleasure and connection with your partner.

Other fundamental aspects include practicing breathwork, meditation, visualizations, and mantras. These elements serve to enhance the union between partners and create a deeper level of intimacy.

The Kama Sutra

The Kama Sutra is an ancient Indian text that dates back around 2,000 years. It's one of the most well-known texts on sexuality and is often referenced when discussing different sexual positions and techniques.

While the Kama Sutra is often associated with Tantra, it should be noted that it is not purely a tantric text. It covers a wide range of subjects related to love and pleasure, including grooming, attraction, flirting, kissing, and more.

However, the Kama Sutra does provide guidance on various sexual positions, techniques, and rituals meant to enhance pleasure and connection between partners. These include positions that allow for deeper penetration, stimulate erogenous zones, and create a sense of intimacy and trust.

Yoni Massage

Yoni massage is a tantric practice that focuses on intimate touch and stimulation of the yoni, or female genitalia. Yoni is a Sanskrit word that translates to "sacred space" or "temple," and the practice of yoni massage honors the sacredness of the female body.

The purpose of yoni massage isn't solely for sexual pleasure but to create a space for healing, connection, and intimacy between partners. The massage is generally performed by the male partner on the female partner, but it can also be practiced between same-sex partners or with the aid of a professional practitioner.

Yoni massage is typically performed after a period of connection and relaxation, using massage oil to hydrate and stimulate the skin. The goal is not to achieve orgasm, but to allow the energy to flow freely through the body and connect with the partner on a deeper level.

Techniques for Increasing Pleasure and Connection

There are various techniques that couples can use to increase pleasure and connection during tantric sex. One technique is to focus on the breath, syncing it with your partner's breathing. This breathing exercise helps cultivate a deeper level of intimacy and synchronization between the two partners.

Another technique is to practice eye-gazing. This involves looking deeply into your partner's eyes and allowing yourself to become fully present and vulnerable. Eye-gazing is a powerful way to deepen intimacy and connection during sex.

Sexual positions also play a significant role in enhancing pleasure and connection during tantric sex. Some positions that are commonly used in tantric sex include the Yab-Yum position, where the female sits on top of the male partner and both partners are face to face, and the Lotus position, where both partners sit with their legs crossed facing each other.

Benefits of Sexual Practices in Achieving Higher States of Consciousness

One of the main goals of tantric sex practices is to achieve higher states of consciousness, which can lead to spiritual growth and enlightenment. By cultivating a deep level of intimacy and connection with a partner, individuals can tap into the divine energy that flows through all things.

Tantric sex practices can also have physical and emotional benefits, such as reducing stress levels, increasing feelings of pleasure and satisfaction, and promoting overall well-being. When we allow ourselves to be fully present during sex, we can let go of our inhibitions and connect with our bodies on a deeper level, leading to a sense of inner peace and contentment.

Additionally, tantric sex practices can help couples heal from past traumas or overcome sexual issues. By creating a safe and nurturing space for intimacy and connection, partners can work together to overcome any challenges they may be facing in their sexual relationship and strengthen their bond.

The Importance of Consent

While tantric sex practices can be highly satisfying and beneficial, it's crucial to emphasize the importance of consent. All partners involved should give enthusiastic and continual consent throughout the entire sexual encounter.

Tantra emphasizes the importance of approaching sex with a deep level of respect, compassion, and empathy. It's important to prioritize your partner's needs and desires, and to communicate openly and honestly about your own wants and boundaries.

Consent is an ongoing process that should be continually assessed and communicated throughout the entire sexual encounter. All parties involved should feel safe, comfortable, and fully empowered to express their desires and boundaries.

In conclusion, tantric sex practices offer numerous benefits for individuals and couples looking to deepen their intimacy and connection. By emphasizing the importance of mindfulness, awareness, and respect, individuals can tap into a deeper level of consciousness and spiritual growth, while also experiencing physical and emotional benefits. However, it's crucial to prioritize consent and communication throughout the entire sexual encounter, creating a safe and nurturing space for exploration and connection. Remember to approach sex with respect, compassion, and empathy, and prioritize your partner's needs and desires while being honest about your own. Through these practices, individuals can experience a profound sense of pleasure and satisfaction, while strengthening their bond with their partner.

Chapter 6

Incorporating Tantra into Your Relationship

Incorporating Tantra into your relationship can enhance intimacy, strengthen communication, and deepen your spiritual connection with your partner. In this chapter, we'll explore ways to approach discussing Tantra with your partner, how to introduce it into your intimate relationship, and how to build trust and communication through Tantric practices.

How to Approach Discussing Tantra with Your Partner

Bringing up the topic of Tantric sex with your partner can be challenging, especially if one or both of you have limited experience with Tantra. Here are some tips on how to approach the subject with your partner.

Begin by expressing your desire to enhance your connection with your partner.

Start by expressing your desire to explore new ways to connect with your partner on a deeper level. Tell them that you're open to exploring new ways of bringing intimacy and spiritual growth into your relationship.

Share information about Tantra and its benefits.

Provide your partner with a basic understanding of Tantric principles, such as mindfulness, presence, and sexual spirituality. Offer them resources, such as books or articles, to learn more about the practice and its potential benefits for your relationship.

Be open about your own apprehensions and concerns.

Cheryl Bach

If you have doubts or concerns about introducing Tantra into your relationship, talk about them openly and honestly with your partner. Encourage them to do the same, and work together to address any issues or reservations that either of you might have.

Set boundaries and expectations for your exploration.

Agree on boundaries and expectations for exploring Tantric practices in your relationship. Create an environment of mutual respect, honesty, and safety, and ensure that both partners feel empowered to communicate their needs and desires.

Be patient and understanding.

Remember that introducing Tantra into your relationship can be a process that takes time, patience, and understanding. Be patient with your partner and allow them to become comfortable with the idea of exploring Tantric practices at their own pace.

Introducing Tantra into Your Intimate Relationship

Now that you've discussed the concept of Tantra with your partner, it's time to begin to explore how to introduce it into your intimate relationship.

Begin with mindfulness practices.

Start by incorporating mindfulness practices into your daily routine as a couple. This can include simple practices such as meditation before you go to bed, practicing deep breathing exercises together, or taking mindful walks in nature.

Share Tantra-inspired experiences.

Explore sensual activities together such as an intimate massage with essential oils, taking a sensual bath or shower together, or enjoying a slow, sensual dance together. These activities can help you both to be present and mindful of each other, deepening your connection and intimacy.

Experiment with Tantric sex techniques.

As you become more comfortable with mindfulness and sensual activities, you can begin to experiment with Tantric sex techniques. These techniques can include prolonged foreplay, conscious touch, tantric breathing, and exploring multiple orgasms. Remember to always communicate with your partner, listen to their needs and desires, and set boundaries beforehand.

Explore Tantric rituals together.

Tantric rituals can be a powerful way to deepen spiritual connection and intimacy in your relationship. These can include practices such as tantric puja, where you perform rituals and chants together, or yoni (vaginal) massage for women and lingam (penis) massage for men. It's important to approach these rituals with respect, openness, and a willingness to learn and grow together.

Incorporate Tantric principles into your everyday life.

Tantra isn't just about what you do in the bedroom; it's a way of life that extends beyond your intimate relationship. Incorporate Tantric principles into your everyday life by practicing self-care, mindfulness, and compassion for yourself and others. You can also explore spiritual practices such as yoga or meditation together as a couple.

Building Trust and Communication in Your Relationship through Tantra

Tantra can be a powerful tool for building trust and communication in your relationship. Here are some ways to explore these benefits:

Practice active listening.

One of the key elements of Tantra is being present and fully engaged with your partner. Practice active listening by giving your partner your full attention, validating their feelings, and empathizing with their experiences. This helps to build trust and deepen your connection.

Practice non-judgment.

Another important Tantric principle is non-judgment. When you approach your partner and their experiences without judgment, you create a space for openness, honesty, and vulnerability.

Explore your desires and boundaries.

Tantric practices require a high degree of communication and trust. As you explore Tantric techniques, make sure you have clear communication about your boundaries, desires, and limitations. This creates a safe space where both partners feel supported and respected.

Build intimacy through eye contact.

One of the most effective ways to build intimacy in your relationship is through eye contact. As you explore Tantric practices, use eye contact to connect with your partner on a deeper level. This helps to create a sense of trust, intimacy, and presence.

Use touch to deepen your connection.

Touch is a powerful tool for deepening your connection and building trust in your relationship. Experiment with different types of touch, such as slow caresses or holding each other close, and see how it impacts your intimacy.

Embracing Spirituality in Your Relationship through Tantra

Tantra is often associated with spirituality, and can be used as a way to deepen your connection with yourself, your partner, and the universe. Here are some ways to embrace spirituality in your relationship through Tantra:

Practice gratitude.

Gratitude is an essential element of spiritual practice. Take time every day to express gratitude for each other and for the blessings in your life. This helps to cultivate a sense of abundance and positivity in your relationship.

Connect with nature.

Nature is a powerful spiritual force that can help you connect with a deeper sense of self and the universe. Spend time together in nature, whether it's hiking, picnicking, or simply taking a walk. This helps to ground you and create a sense of calm and balance.

Meditate together.

Meditation is a powerful tool for connecting with your inner self and the universe. Meditate together as a couple to deepen your connection and create a sense of shared spiritual practice.

Incorporate mantras into your practice.

Mantras are powerful phrases or sounds that help to focus your mind and connect with the universe. Choose a mantra that resonates with both of you and incorporate it into your Tantric practice.

Explore the chakras.

The chakras are energy centers in the body that are associated with different aspects of physical, emotional, and spiritual well-being. Exploring the chakras together can help you deepen your understanding of each other and connect on a more spiritual level. You can incorporate chakra-balancing practices into your Tantric practice, such as focusing on a specific chakra during meditation or using affirmations to balance the energy in each chakra.

Overall, Tantra can be an incredibly powerful tool for deepening your connection with your partner and exploring new levels of intimacy and spirituality. By approaching it with openness, curiosity, and respect for each other's boundaries, you can create a deeply fulfilling and meaningful relationship with your partner.

Chapter 7

Advanced Tantra Techniques

In the previous chapters, we explored the basic techniques and principles of Tantric sex. Now, it's time to take your practice to the next level with some advanced techniques that can help you deepen your connection and experience even greater pleasure and bliss.

Advanced Techniques

The Yab-Yum Position

The Yab-Yum position is one of the most iconic Tantric sex positions, and for good reason. It allows for deep penetration and intimate eye contact, creating a sense of union with your partner that transcends the physical. To try the Yab-Yum position, have your partner sit cross-legged with their back straight, while you straddle them facing them, wrapping your legs around them. You can then synchronize your breath and rock together in a slow, rhythmic motion.

The Sahaja Position

The Sahaja position is another advanced Tantric sex position that involves deep penetration and intense eye contact. To try the Sahaja position, have your partner lay on their back with their legs open, while you sit between their legs facing them. You can then wrap your arms around their thighs and look deeply into their eyes while you penetrate them deeply.

Controlled Breathing

Breath control is an important aspect of Tantric sex, and mastering it can lead to even greater levels of pleasure and intimacy. Try synchronized breathing exercises with your partner, where you inhale and exhale together, focusing on the sensation of your breath moving in and out of your body. As you approach orgasm, try holding your breath briefly to build up tension, before releasing it and letting the orgasm wash over you.

Sensory Deprivation

Sensory deprivation is an intensive Tantric technique that can help you experience heightened sensations and deeper levels of connection with your partner. It involves temporarily depriving one or more senses, such as sight or hearing, to enhance the others. To try sensory deprivation, blindfold or deafen your partner, then focus on exploring their body with your remaining senses. You'll be able to feel every touch, taste every sensation, and hear every breath, creating a world of sensual pleasure that you share exclusively with each other.

Chakra Healing

In Tantric sex, each chakra is associated with different aspects of physical, emotional, and spiritual well-being. By focusing on healing and balancing these energy centers through Tantric sex, you can deepen your connection with your partner and elevate your practice to new heights of intimacy and pleasure. You can explore chakra healing by focusing on a specific chakra during sex, incorporating affirmations and visualization techniques, or using specific sex positions that stimulate certain chakras. For example, the Root Chakra is associated with grounding and security, while the Heart Chakra is associated with love and connection.

Navigating Challenges and Setbacks in Your Practice

As with any spiritual practice, you may encounter challenges and setbacks along the way. These could include physical or emotional pain, difficulties communicating with your partner, or feeling stuck in your practice. It's important to listen to your body and your intuition and take a break if necessary. Remember that Tantric sex is about mutual respect and communication, so don't be afraid to ask for what you need or express your concerns to your partner.

Advancing Your Spiritual and Intimate Connection

As you continue with your Tantric sex practice, remember that it's about more than just physical pleasure. It's about deepening your spiritual and emotional connection with your partner.

Here are some tips for advancing your connection:

Communication: Continue to communicate openly and honestly with your partner about your desires, needs, and boundaries.

Intention: Set an intention before each Tantra session to ensure that you're both aligned spiritually and emotionally.

Practice: Make time for regular Tantric sex practice and incorporate new techniques and positions to keep things fresh and exciting.

Play: Remember to have fun with your partner and don't take your practice too seriously.

Gratitude: Express gratitude towards your partner for sharing this intimate and spiritual journey with you.

In conclusion, advanced Tantra techniques can elevate your practice to new levels of intimacy and pleasure. By continuing to communicate openly with your partner, setting intentions, incorporating new techniques, and expressing gratitude, you can deepen your spiritual and emotional connection and experience a greater sense of well-being. Remember to approach your practice with an open mind, honoring your body and your partner at every step. With patience, dedication, and mutual respect, you can

Cheryl Bach

discover the true magic and transformative power of Tantric
sex.

Chapter 8

Maintaining Your Tantric Practice

Congratulations on embarking on your journey to elevate your spiritual and intimate connection through Tantric sex. As you continue to practice Tantra, it's important to find ways to incorporate it into your daily life and maintain the connection with your partner.

Tips for Continuing to Practice Tantra in Your Everyday Life

In this chapter, we'll share tips for continuing your Tantric practice, incorporating it into long-term relationships, and navigating changes in your relationship through continued practice.

Cheryl Bach

Create a Daily Ritual

To maintain your Tantric practice, it's important to make it a part of your daily routine. Set aside time each day for meditation, self-reflection, and practice with your partner. This can be as simple as starting and ending your day with a few minutes of focused breathing together or incorporating Tantric exercises during your morning yoga routine.

Practice Mindful Touch

Another way to maintain your Tantric practice is by practicing mindful touch. This means being completely present and focused on the sensations of touch, while letting go of any distracting thoughts. When you touch your partner, do so with a soft, gentle touch, using your hands and fingers to explore their body. Take the time to notice how their skin feels against yours, the warmth of their body, and the way they respond to your touch. Be mindful of your own sensations and emotions as well, and communicate openly with your partner about what feels good and what doesn't.

Incorporate Sound Healing

Sound healing is a powerful way to enhance your Tantric practice, as it can help deepen your connection with your partner and promote overall emotional and physical well-being. There are several ways you can incorporate sound healing into your practice, such as using music, chanting, or sacred instruments like gongs or crystal bowls. Experiment with different types of sound and find what resonates with you and your partner. During your Tantric sessions, allow the sound vibrations to wash over you and deepen your connection. You can also incorporate sound healing into your daily practice by listening to calming music while meditating or doing yoga.

Share Your Feelings and Desires

Cheryl Bach

Communication is a crucial aspect of any intimate relationship, especially when practicing Tantra. Take the time to talk with your partner about your feelings, desires, and needs, and encourage them to do the same. This open communication will deepen your connection and help prevent misunderstandings or miscommunications from getting in the way of your practice.

Embrace Change and Growth

As your relationship and practice evolve over time, it's important to embrace change and growth. Tantric sex is an intimate form of practice that requires ongoing effort and dedication, and as you continue along this journey, it's natural for your practice to change and grow. Be open to new experiences and challenges, and don't be afraid to experiment with different techniques or approaches to deepen your connection with your partner.

Practice Self-Love and Self-Care

Finally, it's important to remember that your Tantric practice is about more than just your connection with your partner – it's also about your own personal growth and well-being. Take the time to practice self-love and self-care, whether that means taking a relaxing bath, getting a massage, or simply spending some time alone. By nurturing your own physical and emotional health, you'll be better equipped to deepen your connection with your partner and maintain your Tantric practice over the long term.

How to Incorporate Tantra into Long-Term Relationships

Incorporating Tantra into a long-term relationship requires communication and a shared desire to explore new things in your sexual relationship. Communication and setting common goals and expectations are essential. Take the time to set aside moments for intimacy and practice. This could be through meditation, yoga, or other mind-body rituals. Experiment with new Tantric sex positions, sensual touch techniques, and breathing exercises. And most importantly, approach everything with an open and curious mindset.

Navigating Changes in Your Relationship through Continued Practice

Relationships undergo changes over time, and it is important to navigate these changes with an open mind and continued practice. Celebrate changes as they come your way, embrace them with an open heart. Maintain communication and stay committed to the practice that brought you together. As you navigate changes, recognize that your Tantric practice is a tool that can help you connect with one another and deepen intimacy. Mindfulness practices can help you stay present in the moment and navigate any emotional turmoil that may arise as a result of change. Remember, inconsistency is a natural part of change. Continue to practice and honor your commitment to yourself and each other. By using Tantra as a way to explore and embrace changes, you can help your relationship evolve and grow stronger over time.

In conclusion, maintaining your Tantric practice requires effort, dedication, and an open mind. By creating a daily ritual, practicing mindful touch, incorporating sound healing, sharing your feelings and desires, embracing change and growth, and practicing self-love and self-care, you can deepen your connection with your partner and continue to evolve your Tantric practice over time. Remember that the journey is just as important as the destination, and by staying committed to your practice and each other, you can experience the transformative power of Tantra in all aspects of your life.

Cheryl Bach

Chapter 9

Conclusion

Throughout this comprehensive guide on how to practice Tantra's intimate form of sex and Tantric sex techniques to enhance your connection with your partner, we have discussed the principles and practices of Tantra that can help deepen intimacy between you and your partner.

First, we delved into the concept of mindfulness and how it can connect you to ourselves and our partners. We then explored the various Tantric sex positions, breathing techniques, and methods that can ignite sexual energy and allow for deeper connection and intimacy between partners.

We also discussed how incorporating visualizations, sound healing, and sharing feelings and desires in Tantric practice can help couples cultivate stronger emotional bonds that extend beyond the bedroom. The book has also covered essential techniques on how to overcome obstacles like sexual dysfunction, negative emotions, and physical discomfort.

It's important to remember that the key to incorporating Tantric practice into your sexual relationship is communication, honesty, and mutual respect. Tantra is an ongoing practice that requires consistent effort from both partners, and it's essential not to rush the process or force any aspects of the practice.

As we wrap up this book on Tantric sex, we'd like to leave you with some final thoughts and encouragement to continue exploring the world of Tantra and how it can enhance your relationship with your partner.

Firstly, always remember that a Tantric practice is unique to each individual and couple. What works for one person or relationship may not work for another. However, with patience, an open mind, and commitment, you can find what works best for you and your partner.

Secondly, communication and mindfulness are the pillars of any successful Tantric practice. Cultivate a deep connection with yourself first, and then use your Tantric practice to deepen your connection with your partner. Practice active listening, share your feelings and desires with one another, and approach each practice with an open and curious mindset.

Thirdly, be patient with yourself and your partner. Deepening sexual intimacy and emotional connection takes time, and it's normal to encounter obstacles along the way. Don't be discouraged if you don't see immediate results or if things don't go as planned. Embrace the journey and enjoy the process of exploring new things together.

Lastly, we encourage you to keep practicing. Tantra is a lifelong practice that can continually evolve and deepen. Make room for intimacy and connection in your life and relationship, and use your Tantric tools to enhance them. By doing so, you can experience deeper levels of pleasure and connection with your partner while cultivating a stronger relationship that extends beyond the bedroom.

www.ingramcontent.com/pod-product-compliance
Lightning Source LLC
Chambersburg PA
CBHW050829250726

48653CB00006B/2518